Mindfulness Secrets

90 *Ways in 90 Days*

By José Johnson

©2019 José Johnson

All rights reserved. No portion of this book may be reproduced, stored in a retrieval system, or transmitted in any form or by any means - electronic, mechanical, photocopy, recording, scanning, or other, - except for brief quotations in critical reviews or articles, without prior written permission of the publisher.

Table of Contents

Introduction 5
But First, What Is Mindfulness? 7
Setting Up Your Mindfulness Practice 10
   1. Decide which area of your life is most in need of your attention. 12
   2. Intentionally create your day. 13
   3. Pick a card - any card. 14
   4. Alarms and reminders 15
   5. Set a trigger 15
Tools For Your Toolbox 17
   6. Just breathe. 18
   7. Stand Up Sit Down 19
   8. Mindfulness Meditation 19
   9. Body Scan 20
   10. Square Breathing 20
Mindful Movement 22
   11. Tai Chi 23
   12. Qigong 23
   13. Yoga 24
   14. Mindful Muscles 24
   15. Take A Swim 25
   16. Take A Hike 25
Use Your Senses 26

17. Mindful Eating 27
18. Listen To The Music 27
19. See The Rainbow 28
20. Smooth As Silk 28
21. Aromatherapy 29
22. Pretend You're Daredevil 29

Mindfulness In Our Relationships 30
23. Mindful Listening 31
24. Give A Hug 32
25. I Want Your Sex 32

Mindfulness and Money 34
26. Mindful Spending 35
27. Mindful Earning 35
28. Mindful Giving 37

Watch Your Mouth 38
29. Sweet Talk 39
30. If You Can't Say Anything Nice 39
31. Zip It! 39

Mindfulness And Technology 41
32. Brain Entrainment 42
33. Measuring Devices 44
34. Mindfulness Apps 45
35. And Speaking Of Apps 45

A Spiritual Approach To Mindfulness 47

- 36. And Now We Pray ... 48
- 37. Om mani padme huh? ... 48

An Ocean Of Possibilities ... 51
- 38. Time To Hit The Showers ... 52
- 39. You Need A Cold Shower ... 52
- 40. Floating ... 53

Pen And Paper ... 54
- 41. Journaling ... 55
- 42. Keep A Gratitude Journal ... 55
- 43. Do A Mind Dump ... 56
- 31 Daily Affirmations ... 58

14 Random Opportunities ... 63

About The Author ... 70

INTRODUCTION

Why 90 ways? Why 90 days?

Well, first of all, it sounds kind of cool, right?

I mean would you be interested in a book called "Numerous Ways in Approximately 56-66 Days?" Doesn't evoke the same image.

So where do those numbers come from?

First, according to research on the power of mindfulness practice, it takes approximately eight weeks of regular practice to create measurable change to the brain. That means we need at least 56 days to hardwire change.

Second, in order to achieve the best results, mindfulness practice should become a daily habit, and according to research, it takes an average of 66 days to establish a new habit.

So why 90 days? By shooting for 90 days you get a few extra days cushion to lock in the benefits and establish your new habit.

Over the course of this book, I will share with you a collection of strategies and techniques to create your own daily mindfulness practice routines.

Some, like meditation, will be common knowledge. However, some of the ideas in this book might catch you off guard.

The trick is to find the strategies (how you set up your practice) and the techniques (what you practice) to create a routine that is effective, enjoyable and sustainable for you.

Once you get started, the goal is to remain consistent in your practice for 90 days. It's not important that you do the same thing every day or for the same length of time every session. Just do your best to do a little every day without fail.

BUT FIRST, WHAT IS MINDFULNESS?

Here's a little experiment I want you to try right now.

Stand in front of an object like a picture, a light, your computer screen..whatever.

First, focus on that object.

Now take one hand and place it in your field of vision between you and the object.

Depending on what most captures your attention, either the first object will be clear and your hand blurry, or vice versa.

Now take your other hand and place it in your field of vision in front of the first hand.

What happened this time? What is clear and what is blurry?

Now try to shift your focus between the objects.

First, focus on the closest hand and notice what happens to your other hand and the object.

Now focus on the middle hand. Then focus on the far object.

Did you notice that as your attention is drawn to one object the others become fuzzy?

That's what we do with mindfulness.

Mindfulness is not about having no thoughts, it's about focusing on a single thought or idea. And that idea is the present.

Think about the previous exercise, and let's say that the object that is furthest away is your future, the one in the middle is your present and the one closest to you is your past. The practice of mindfulness would be to focus our attention on that middle object or idea of the present so that the future and past become less dominant in our perceptions.

Not focusing on the present is one of the biggest problems that we face. Many of us are either too focused on our past or too concerned about what our future might look like.

I am in no way saying that these things should be ignored, but when we are obsessed with the past we stop growing and are often plagued by guilt and depression. When we become obsessed with the future we create fear and anxiety.

When we are trapped between the two we feel stress. By that I mean that we feel our future fears pulling us forward, our past experiences pulling us backwards, and the present moment stuck in the middle of an emotional tug of war.

So how do you break the cycle? The answer is by learning to focus on the present moment. That is what mindfulness does for us.

Being mindful doesn't erase the past, but it can allow you to look at it from a new perspective. Being mindful doesn't mean that you don't plan for the future. Rather it gives you a firm foundation from which to start. Mindfulness is not something abstract and exclusive. It is concrete and inclusive. When you practice mindfulness, the key is to be more of an observer of the present than judge, jury and executioner.

Ultimately our aim should be to live a mindful life, not just practice mindfulness.

SETTING UP YOUR MINDFULNESS PRACTICE

Each of us has the ability to be mindful And just like walking or running, it takes time and practice to improve your skills. The problem is that most people have no idea how and where to start. That's where this book comes in. I want to dispel some of the myths and misconceptions around mindfulness in order to make it easier for you to gain the benefits that you are searching for.

The first myth is that mindfulness practice takes hours a day.

While most research surrounding the benefits of mindfulness used a 20-minute session as the baseline requirement, you can get a near immediate benefit if you know how to maximize your practice.

Let me share a related story with you.

I used to be an international level martial arts competitor. My specialty was Tai Chi. When I was training for the final season of my career, I would often train eight or more hours a day for six days a week. During that period, I achieved tremendous results. However, that intensity of training was not sustainable, and I often felt guilty when I took a day off. When I realized that I could make everything that I did "practice" that my skill level skyrocketed. I didn't have to be in the gym to work on my posture, my balance, my coordination, my focus or my breathing. When I focused on those essential skills in my day-to-day activities, I was constantly practicing. And because I was constantly practicing, I was constantly improving. By creating that mindshift I was able to focus more time on the specific skills I needed to work on instead of the general skills. When I figured out how to go from practicing Tai Chi to living Tai Chi, I improved my results exponentially without having to live in the training hall.

The same applies to mindfulness practice. Creating a dedicated time and place to practice will help you establish a routine. However, your ultimate goal should be to make every moment an opportunity to be mindful.

That being said, you do need to start somewhere.

Following are my ideas for 90 ways to create an effective and manageable approach to creating your personal mindfulness practice routine in 90 days.

1. Decide which area of your life is most in need of your attention.

I have a personalized approach to this called the "Five Pillars of Holistic Wellness." The idea is a result of my study of Chinese martial arts, healing arts, and philosophy.

In Chinese culture there exists a concept called the "Wu Xing" or "Five Phases/Elements." This theory has been used for centuries to explain the relationship and interactions found in nature - everything from the changing of the seasons to the changes in the socio-political climate. There is even an entire method of Chinese medicine devoted to the use of the Five Phases theory to diagnose and treat illness.

The Five Pillars of Holistic Wellness is my way of looking at the relationship of the major parts of life. The pillars support who we are and what we are able to do.

The Five Pillars are:

- Physical Wellness
- Mental Wellness
- Emotional Wellness
- Spiritual Wellness
- Financial Wellness

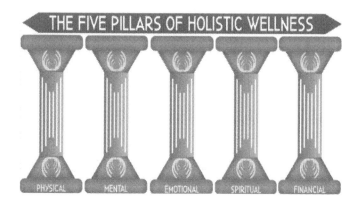

Why holistic? Because life is not simply a series of unrelated events. Every aspect of our lives has an effect on the others. If you want to live your life to its fullest, you need to understand how each part works to support or detract from the others. My method for mindfulness practice incorporates this theory as a way to create clarity of focus. In other words, I consider the Five Pillars of Holistic Wellness to help me figure out which area or areas of my life would best benefit from a little extra mindfulness.

Which pillar of your life do you need to be more mindful of?

2. Intentionally create your day.

Now that you have a clearer idea of which pillar of your life needs a little extra attention, the next step is to create your plan of action...or non action if you are trying to be all Zen.

Take a few moments before you start your day to create a picture in your mind of how you want your day to go. Decide on what practices you want to incorporate. If you want even better results, do this right before going to bed the night before. This will allow your subconscious mind to get an early start on things while you sleep.

I strongly suggest writing down your intentions. Use a journal, a loose sheet of paper, a note card (my favorite) or even on your hand. The process of writing something down adds another layer of mindfulness to the equation, and keeping your written intentions with you and looking at them during the day helps your mind stay on track.

3. Pick a card - any card.

Another way of finding your focus is to let the Universe do it for you.

Take a stack of index cards and write a different mindful intention on each card. Something like smile at everyone you meet or be aware of your posture.

Mix up the pile and pick a card.

Whatever the card says is now your intention for the day.

A more advanced version of this method is to create different decks for different aspects of your practice. One deck for your pillars, one deck for specific techniques and one for the frequency or duration of your practice (once a day, at meals, for 5 minutes, etc.) Pick cards from each deck to create your mindfulness practice for the day.

4. Alarms and reminders.

If you want to engage in your mindfulness practice at a specific time, try setting an alarm or a reminder in your phone.

One of the problems that we face with our reliance on our phones is that we have a Pavlovian response to them. It's hard for us to ignore a beep, chime or buzz. It's the dopamine rush of something new and exciting.

So use it to your favor and set an alarm to remind yourself to be mindful.

5. Set a trigger.

Another way to remind yourself to practice mindfulness is to attach the practice to a trigger event.

Pick an event or location, like when you are brushing your teeth, everytime you are stopped at a traffic light, or whenever you pass by a mirror, as the prompt or trigger to do your practice.

The prompt could also be tied to an upcoming event that you know will be stressful, like making sure you do some type of practice before your Monday morning staff meeting.

Tools For Your Toolbox

Now that you have an idea of how you can create a daily mindfulness practice, you need to have the techniques, the "what" to your how.

The following pages contain the ways you can practice mindfulness. Think of these as the tools in your toolbox. Each of these practices give you a different way to experience mindfulness.Just like you wouldn't use a hammer to tighten a bolt, it's important to have a number of methods available to you so that you can pick the right tool for the job.

So let's start with the basics.

6. Just breathe.

The simplest and most commonly practiced mindfulness method is simply to become aware of your breathing.

Bring your attention to your breath. Focus on the timing. Focus on the "quality" of your breath. Is it smooth and even? Deep? Full?

Don't try to change anything about your breathing (that's later), just pay attention to how you are breathing and how it makes you feel.

The way I like to think about breathing is to imagine you are smelling something that makes you feel good.

One of my fondest memories as a child was when my mother would make fresh baked rolls for the holidays. To this day the smell of bread baking immediately triggers positive emotions.

When you breathe, take in that full deep breath. Savor it. When you release it, you should feel like you want to let out a content sigh.

Always make sure to breathe in through your nose. Depending on when and where you are practicing, you can choose to exhale through either the nose or the mouth.

Deep breathing activates our Parasympathetic Nervous System (PNS) which helps to calm the body.

7. Stand Up Sit Down

Your posture has a great deal to do with your sense of well-being.

A change in how you sit or stand can create a change in how you feel internally, and an internal change often manifests itself in a change of posture.

When we bring our awareness to our posture we can begin to tap into our thoughts and emotions.

8. Mindfulness Meditation

As one of my teachers always said, "Meditation is allowing one thought to represent 10, 000 others." Meditation is not about not thinking. Rather it's about not thinking about what you don't want to think about. It's focusing your mind.

There are a number of ways to approach meditation, and each approach has its own unique benefit. Mindfulness meditation is specific in its approach.

The purpose of mindfulness meditation is to be aware of the present moment, to experience what is happening in you and around you without judgement.

You can use a variety of the tools presented in this book as part of your mindful meditation. The most common are the body scan and square breathing.

9. Body Scan

A body scan involves taking your time to pay attention to how your body feels.

Simply start at the top of your head and use your mind to scan down your body and "check in" with yourself. How does your jaw feel? How do your shoulders feel? Your chest? Your back? Your knees? Your toes?

When you do this process you can either register how every part of your body feels and move on, or you can go back through the scan and try to release any excess tension or pain that your body is holding on to. You can repeat this process as many times as you like or have time for.

If you have trouble falling asleep at night, try doing a body scan as you lie in bed.

10. Square Breathing

Square breathing (or box breathing) is a simple breathing method that can be used as part of your meditation practice.

To do square breathing, you just need to be able to breathe and count to four.

Nothing too crazy so far, right?

Start by taking a deep but relaxed breath for a count of four.

Next gently hold your breath for another count of four.

Now release the breath for another count of four.

Finally hold the exhalation state for another four counts.

And just repeat.

The key to square breathing is that it needs to be extremely relaxed. You don't want to tank up your lungs like you are trying to blow out the candles on your birthday cake. When you hold your breath, it shouldn't feel like you are throwing a tantrum and waiting to turn blue.

If you have problems with your blood pressure, be careful about holding your breath. Make sure that you stay as relaxed as possible. If at any point you start to feel dizzy, stop trying to control your breath. Sit down and go back to your normal respiration pattern until you feel better.

Mindful Movement

While sitting and meditating is a great way to become present, movement should not be overlooked.

11. Tai Chi

Tai Chi Chuan (or Taijiquan) is a popular style of Chinese martial arts. It has been called "meditation in motion" and has been the subject of numerous research studies related to its benefits for physical, cognitive and emotional health.

Unlike most other styles of martial arts, Tai Chi emphasises a much more "laid back" approach to its practice. Tai Chi is generally practiced at a much slower pace than other martial arts. The idea is to become totally aware of the moment - to listen to your body as well as to connect with the intention of your "partner."

The performance of long sequences (forms) require a level of concentration and memory as well as coordination.

12. Qigong

Often confused with Tai Chi, Qigong is another Chinese practice that helps the practitioner enter a mindful state.

Technically, Qigong is a broad category of practices. It literally translates as "energy skill" so anything that helps the practitioner control, develop, or become more aware of their innate energy is a Qigong. Tai Chi is a martial art that has a very strong Qigong component.

In most cases, Qigong methods are much less complicated than Tai Chi in terms of the sequence of movements.

13. Yoga

Yoga is probably the physical activity most often associated with mindfulness. Yoga literally means union. The study of Yogic practices is a way of helping you become unified with yourself, your environment and the universe. While practicing the physical exercises that we commonly call Yoga, you must keep your body, mind, emotions and breath calm and unified.

Yoga requires physical strength, flexibility and balance to create the various postures. And the more complex and challenging the physical postures the more calm, aware and focused the mind has to be.

14. Mindful Muscles

Try this the next time you are at the gym.

Instead of just rushing through your workout and counting reps and sets, slow down and focus on your actions. Become aware of how your entire body is engaged in each exercise, or just focus on the muscle group being worked.

15. Take A Swim

Swimming is another great exercise to use as a mindfulness practice.

When you are swimming, you get the benefits of physical awareness, breath control and the calming effect of being in the water.

16. Take A Hike

Feeling stressed? Take a hike. Or just a walk around the block. Getting up and moving helps to reset our brains. In fact, our brains were designed to solve problems on the run. It's what kept our ancestors from being eaten by all those prehistoric predators. It's also why we instinctively do things like tap our fingers, wiggle our feet, rock in our chair or pace the room when we are trying to solve a complex problem.

By creating a change of scenery, we can begin to create a change in perspective. New things to see and experience create new neural connections. This helps us see our problems in a new light.

USE YOUR SENSES

Our senses are how we connect to the external world. What we see. What we smell. What we taste. What we hear. What we feel.

Our senses pick up millions of bits of information every second - eleven million to be precise. However, our brain only consciously registers 50 bits per second. That means that a lot of stuff is going on beneath our level of awareness.

Here are some ways to pick up on some of the stuff we may have been missing.

17. Mindful Eating

I attended a presentation on how to eat chocolate at a famous chocolate company. In the presentation they talked about how to use your five senses when eating their products, how there is a difference not just in taste but in the look, the smell, the texture, even the sound when you broke the bars apart.

The next time you are enjoying a candy bar, an apple, a cup of coffee or a glass of wine, try engaging all of your senses.

18. Listen To The Music

Being a trumpet player, any time there is a horn playing on a song my mind immediately focuses in on it. It's something I intimately relate to. It's also a skill that I developed after years of having to learn horn parts off a recording.

The next time you listen to music, try focusing your attention on one instrument at a time. Perhaps you focus on the drums or bass. Maybe you listen intently to the lyrics. Listen for the subtleties of the vocalists phrasing, pick out a specific harmony or even listen for the acoustics or effects used in the recording process.

19. See The Rainbow

There is a part of our brain called the Reticular Activating System that helps us to filter out unnecessary information and focus in on what we feel is essential. Generally the RAS works on a subconscious level. However we can choose to directly tap into it. One way is through focusing on color.

Try setting an intention to look for a specific color, like red. Hold this intention as look around, taking note of all the red things that you see. You might be surprised at how many new red things you will suddenly become aware of.

20. Smooth As Silk

Most people know that the fingertips are highly packed with nerve receptors and are our go-to for our sense of touch, but there are other areas of our bodies that are quite sensitive as well.

Try taking objects with different textures (preferably not too rough) and rubbing them on your arm, your shin, your face or across your lips. Notice how the same object can feel different based on the nerves that are stimulated.

21. Aromatherapy

Our sense of smell is quite powerful - not as powerful as a dog's, but still pretty amazing.

One of the more amazing things about smell is it's effect on our memories and emotions.

Try smelling different fragrances and focus on the feelings that they stir up.

22. Pretend You're Daredevil

I'm a bit of a comic book geek, and one of the characters that I used to love was Daredevil. He was blinded as a child but his other senses, particularly his hearing, became heightened.

In reality, we see this occur every day. When one sense is lost or diminished, the other senses pick up the slack. There is even research that shows that the remaining sensory organs can annex the neural real estate that the deprived sense would normally hold.

Try doing things with your eyes closed and "see" how that the level of sensitivity in the rest of your body.

Mindfulness In Our Relationships

It's sometimes too easy for us to take our relationships with others for granted. Our family, friends, co-workers, even ourselves.

Being present when you are interacting with another person is the greatest gift we can give them.

Here are a few ways to practice mindfulness in our relationships.

23. Mindful Listening

Did you ever have a conversation with someone only to find that your mind has wandered and you missed something they said? Perhaps you misinterpreted the meaning of something because you really weren't paying attention.

Are you one of those people who talk over others and don't let people finish their thoughts?

Commit to mindful listening.

Don't interrupt. Let people finish their thoughts.

Don't think about what your response to what they are saying will be while they are talking. Take a moment after they are done to formulate your thoughts.

Don't try to lead the conversation. Allow the other person to steer.

Don't try to interpret what the other person is saying. If you aren't clear, ask or say "so what I'm hearing is…"

Listen longer than you talk. Like the old saying goes, we have two ears and one mouth so we can listen twice as more as we speak.

Don't be distracted. Put down your phone. Turn off the TV. Look and listen to the other person.

24. Give A Hug

Research has indicated that hugs can be beneficial for more than just showing your affection. Hugs can reduce pain, lower blood pressure and reduce stress. A hug of 20 seconds releases oxytocin, sometimes called our bonding hormone, which gives us a sense of safety, security and connection.

So next time you give someone a hug, make it a long one. It's a good idea to make sure you have their permission!

25. I Want Your Sex

If there is ever one time when we should be present, it's during the intimacy of sex.

There are tantric practices that use sex not just for procreation or gratification, but as a method of feeling more connected with yourself, your partner and the universe.

The next time you are with that special someone, be completely present. Focus on the range of sensations that you feel in every part of your body, and not just the ones doing the deed. Become aware of your heartbeat and your breathing and how they coordinate with your partners. Make your connection about listening and responding without words.

Use all of your senses to receive and perceive pleasure.

MINDFULNESS AND MONEY

Money.

Seems that we are either thinking about it too much or not enough.

Money is a tool. It's something that we can use to create a better life for ourselves, a better world for others.

Or, money can become our master. We can become a slave to it. We start to live to serve it as opposed to learning to let it serve us.

So how can you become more mindful of your financial pillar?

Here are a few ideas.

26. Mindful Spending

When you spend money are you mindful of the process?

If you are like most people the answer is probably not.

We tend to spend either recklessly or wracked with guilt, and sometimes the former precedes the latter.

The next time you spend money, and that could be anything from paying your utility bills to buying a new pair of shoes, take a moment to become aware of how you feel before you finalize your transaction.

Do you feel happy? Anxious? Angry? Frustrated?

Now take a moment afterwards. How do you feel now?

Do you feel relieved? Guilty?

By becoming aware of your feelings you will become aware of your relationship with money and your reasons for spending.

27. Mindful Earning

How do you earn your money?

Odds are you have some type of job.

If you are like the vast majority of the workforce you really don't like going to work. The hours are too long. The pay isn't enough. The conditions are poor. The demands are too high. Etc, etc.

But how would being mindful help?

Take a moment to check in with yourself throughout the day. How is your attitude? How is your performance?

If it's not where and how you want it to be, why isn't it?

Is it possible to reframe your situation?

One of the tricks that I like to use is to remind myself what my work is for, both in abstract and concrete terms.

For example, you could remind yourself that your work today could make a difference in someone's life (abstract) or that today's shift will pay your electric bill or pay for your next date night (concrete).

In either case, you shift your reaction from the task to a reason with which you have a stronger positive emotional bond.

28. Mindful Giving

Charity is an act that should come from the heart, but do you ever stop to think about how you feel? Be a mindful giver, not just a cheerful giver.

The next time you perform a charitable act, pay attention to how you feel before, during and after. Do you sense a shift?

Also try comparing a relatively small gesture (like leaving your spare change in the donation box by the cash register) to a larger one (like donating $100 to your favorite charity.) Is there a difference? What was it?

You can also try this with different types of charities to see which ones give you the most "bang for your buck."

Watch Your Mouth

How often do you speak without thinking?

The words we speak are the manifestations of the thoughts we think. Make sure you are speaking properly and that you are using the right words in the right way.

To quote Thich Nhat Hanh:

"Before you speak, understand the person you are speaking to. Consider each word carefully before you say anything, so that your speech is "Right" in both form and content."

29. Sweet Talk

Do you encourage or compliment others? If not, you really should. Giving someone a sincere compliment or encouraging word can make both of you feel better.

Make it a point to give at least one compliment to everyone you speak to for a day and see what a difference it makes.

30. If You Can't Say Anything Nice

If our words of encouragement do wonders for ourselves and others, what about our negative talk?

You might be very surprised how many times a day you make negative statements. Whether it's gossip or complaining about your work, the weather or politics, it's easy to get caught up in a downward spiral of negative thoughts.

See how long you can go without making a negative statement.

31. Zip It!

If you really want a challenge, see how long you can go without speaking. And no, while you're sleeping doesn't count.

Keep your thoughts to yourself. Having an extended solitary conversation could allow you to discover things about yourself that you didn't know, or that you were trying to ignore.

Mindfulness And Technology

We live in a world of rapidly developing technology. The purpose of technology is fundamentally to make our lives easier. Sometimes it accomplishes that at a fairly steep cost - and I'm not talking about the cost of the latest smartphone.

Here are a few ways that we can use technology to assist us in our mindfulness practice and a few ways that we need to be very careful of.

32. Brain Entrainment

Because of the electrical nature of your brain, your neural activity can be measured, and one of the types of measurement is something called brainwaves.

According to Webster's Dictionary, brainwaves (or neural oscillations) are defined as "rhythmic fluctuations of voltage between parts of the brain resulting in the flow of an electric current."

Scientists have discovered five basic ranges at which our brains function. Each range correlates with a specific mental state.

Here's the breakdown:

- Delta (0.5 Hz-4 Hz): This is deep sleep
- Theta (4.5Hz-8Hz): This is when you are drowsy or just falling asleep.
- Alpha (8.5 Hz-12Hz): This is when you are relaxed but alert.
- Beta (12.5 Hz-30 Hz): This is when you are highly alert and focused
- Gamma (40 Hz): This state is related to high levels of creativity.

We naturally cycle through the different wave states during the course of a day.

However many people find themselves stuck in the beta state.

Delta? You hit this one when you are zonked out for the night.

Theta and alpha (and sometimes gamma) are the states that meditators want to hit.

But how do you do that?

Well, traditional meditation trains your brain to focus it's thoughts to slow down from the high beta 'monkey mind' to the slower, more chill alpha and theta ranges, but that takes time and dedication.

What if you could train your brain quicker? That's where brain entrainment comes in.

Simply put, brain entrainment uses the process that physicists call entrainment to coax your brain to change frequencies. Entrainment is the process by which one vibrational frequency causes other objects to sync up. With brain entrainment you typically listen to a recording that plays a specific frequency - like 8 beats per second to reach a Theta wave state.
The theory is that because of the entrainment effect, listening to this frequency will make the brain shift gears to mirror the sound you are listening to.

From a mindfulness stand point, brain entrainment technologies can be used to reduce the amount of time it takes to move from a more alert state to a more meditative state.

There are a number of companies that create various types of brain entrainment recordings. While empirical evidence is not conclusive, many people swear by them. I personally use them from time to time and have found them useful in my personal practice.

33. Measuring Devices

While brain entrainment is a way of using external stimuli to change your brainwaves, there are devices that help you to monitor those changes.

Brainwaves are generally monitored with high cost machines like EEG's or fMRI's. Devices that the average (and even above average) person could not afford to keep in their meditation room.

Enter home measuring devices.

In the 70's, biofeedback was "discovered" and at that time several devices (some legit, some bogus) were created as ways to measure what was going on in the brain. Like most things, biofeedback fell out of fashion.

Recently devices like the Muse have become popular.

The Muse works on a very similar format to earlier biofeedback mechanisms. Small contact pads measure changes in the voltage of the skin around your head. The Muse sensor sends the data to a connected app that lets you know how "Zen" you are through feedback in the form of tweeting birds and bubbling brooks. The calmer the sounds, the calmer your mind. The more your mind wanders, the more chaotic the sounds become. I have used The Muse as well and find it a great device to play with and to have in your mindfulness toolbox..or toy box as the case may be.

34. Mindfulness Apps

Yep. There's an app for that.

Actually there are thousands of mindfulness-based apps with more being produced every day.

So how do they work? Each one is a little different, but most have some combination of timed, guided meditations, relaxing sounds and notifications.

The prices range from free to not so cheap, but for people who need a little coaching, they are certainly worth the investment.

35. And Speaking Of Apps

Put down your phone and slowly back away.

One of the best ways to stay present is to put down your portable device.

We live in the information age. There is more information being generated than at any point in our history. In fact, 90% of all of the available data in the world was created in the past two years. The scary part is that we have near instantaneous access to that information through our mobile devices.

It's easy to get sucked down the information vortex. There is so much to learn. To top it off, the algorithms used by companies like Google and Facebook make sure that for every topic we show interest in, we will receive "suggestions" for similar content. If you look up the best way to clean up your cat's litter, you will probably be urged to enter the never ending black hole of funny cat videos from which there is no escape.

Each time you experience something new, your "brain-tender" gives you a big shot of dopamine followed by a cocktail of other 'feel good' neurotransmitters. You feel good, and you lose track of time. Try as you might, you can't pull yourself away, and in large part because the preview for the next video starts before the end of the current video. You aren't given a moment to rest.

Give yourself an information break. Put down the phone and enjoy a few moments without the steady stream of digital information.

A Spiritual Approach To Mindfulness

Our spiritual pillar is all about our connection to something greater than us.

For some of us, it may be God, while for others Allah or Buddha or Shiva. Perhaps you prefer The Dao or The Universe.

Whatever you believe in, we are connected to all things, and every human being has a drive to feel connected with that something in order to find answers to the great existential questions of "who am I" and what is my purpose?" However, our ability to discover those answers is often clouded by the busyness of our physical existence.

In order to better hear the answers, we need to quiet the mind and tune in to the higher frequencies of our personal higher power.

36. And Now We Pray

According to the Cambridge Dictionary, prayer is "the act or ceremony of speaking to God or a god, especially to express thanks, to ask for help, or the words used in this act."

Notice these key words: Act. Speak.. Express thanks. Ask for help.

In other words, prayer is basically a conversation, and I have already given you some tips on mindful conversations. Most people never hear the answer to their prayers because they never shut up long enough to hear it.

Try approaching your prayers as an opportunity to listen for an answer. You could be surprised at what you hear.

37. Om mani padme huh?

The use of mantras is often connected with meditation, and since for many people mindfulness and meditation have become synonymous, they think you have to use a mantra.

As I've already explained, mindfulness and meditation are not the same thing, although we can use meditation to improve our mindfulness.

So what is a mantra, and how do you use it?

Mantra literally means "mind tool" or "tool of thought." It's a way to get the mind focused. The most common mantras are from ancient Sanskrit and are believed to have psychological and spiritual powers.

Believe it or not, there is power in the words we use. Research has shown that the use of a mantra helps to override default-mode network (DMN) distractions. The DMN is located in your medial prefrontal cortex and is the part of the brain that activates when you analyze the past, plan for the future or think about yourself and other people. Research has shown how this area of the brain activates when we are doing a task that we don't need to consciously focus on, like driving, and shifts our attention from the current external environment to our internal dialog.

Sanskrit mantras are not the only "mind tools" that work. Research has shown that mentally repeating "echad", the Hebrew word for one, also provided a calming of the mind.

Does it matter what word or words you say in a mantra? That depends on who you ask. What I can tell you is that there are certain words or phrases that have an emotional valence to them. They are power words.Those words are different for every person.

I can also tell you that certain words have a particular psychoacoustic nature. Psychoacoustics is the study of how sound creates a physiological and psychological effect. It's why happy songs don't use diminished or augmented chords and why the sound someone makes when they are in pain is the same no matter the language.

If you chant the word "Om" you will feel the vibration in a different resonant cavity of the body (the head) as opposed to "Ah" (the throat), and the vibrations in these different spots will create a different feeling.

If you want to create a mantra, make sure that the words have a strong emotional connection for you and for the state you want to be in.

AN OCEAN OF POSSIBILITIES

Water.

Approximately 71% of the Earth is covered with water. Up to 60% of the adult human body is water. Your brain and heart are 73% water. Your lungs are about 83%.

With so much water around us and in us it seems that taking a mindfulness cue from water could be a refreshing change of pace.

38. Time To Hit The Showers

Have you ever wondered why you feel so relaxed or get those sudden flashes on inspiration when you take a warm shower? When we take warm showers our brains start to enter the theta state, that relaxed state where our brains most often experience "flow" or "being in the zone."

The next time you take a nice warm shower, be mindful of the stress and tension being washed away and observe how your creativity starts to shine through.

39. You Need A Cold Shower

I know. Sounds like tourture. However, more and more people are singing the praises of taking cold showers.

Cold showers will obviously increase your circulation and wake up your nerve endings, but research has shown that cold showers can increase the production of noradrenaline, the key neurotransmitter responsible for fighting off depression. Cold showers also increase blood levels of glutathione and decrease levels of uric acid which lead to a state of relaxation. When you take a cold shower you also become very aware of your breathing, and that awareness forces you to take deeper breaths.

So, clear your mind and save your hot water.

40. Floating

The use of sensory deprivation tanks is making a comeback. Float tanks (as they are now called) are enclosed pods filled with salt water that allows you to freely float so that your body can rest and recuperate. They are extremely popular with elite-level athletes as part of their recovery and rehabilitation processes.

When floating, you can completely shut yourself off from the world which allows you to be more present with yourself.

Pen And Paper

Our thoughts are like kids. Sometimes they just want to be heard.

But sometimes you don't particularly want or need to share your thoughts with anyone but yourself.

Here are a few tips to give your thoughts acknowledgement.

41. Journaling

Journaling is a great way to bring your thoughts to life. It is also a great way to help you organize and make sense of your situations and experiences.

Writing relies mainly on left brain functions which allows the creativity centers in the right side to find new solutions to any problem you are experiencing.

There is no need to worry about grammar and spelling. Journaling is just a way of bringing your thoughts to life.

Try writing about a situation from an outside perspective. Become the observer. Doing this allows you to detach from the situation and see things from a point of view that is not as clouded by emotions.

42. Keep A Gratitude Journal

A gratitude journal is a variation of journaling. The focus on this process is, you guessed it, expressing your gratitude.

Sit down and record all the things that you have to be grateful for. This could be an accounting for your entire life or just as it relates to a specific situation.

This is an especially powerful tool to use when dealing with a difficult situation in your life - like illness, financial problems or relationship woes.

Why? Because you have to engage both sides of your brain. The left side is busy writing and your right side is actively searching for and creating new narratives to describe your situation.

As you become aware of the new perspective, your mind is able to basically rewrite your vision of the past so that it supports your current positive feelings.

43. Do A Mind Dump

A mind dump is an extreme version of journaling.

Remember that fact about the 11,000,000 bits of information that we process every second? While our conscious mind registers only 50 of those bits in that second, over the course of the entire day, we process around 4,000,000 bits of information. Where does that information go?

Think about your brain like the photo gallery on your phone. Odds are it is full of things that seemed important enough to document at the time but right now are just hogging up precious memory.

As I said before, thoughts often just want to be recognized so doing a brain dump may be the thing to do when you need absolute clarity.

To do a brain dump sit down with a blank piece of paper and a pen or pencil.

Close your eyes and take a deep breath.

Open your eyes as you exhale and just start writing.

Write everything that comes into your mind.

Just like with journaling, grammar and spelling don't count. And neither does penmanship. This is not about recording your thoughts, it's about releasing your thoughts.

Keep writing until you can't think of another thing to write.

When you are done, either throw away or burn the paper.

Your mind should now be clear from the clutter of excess thoughts, and you can focus on the present moment.

31 Daily Affirmations

Affirmations are another great way to collapse the past and future into the present moment.

Affirmations are similar to mantras on the surface. Mantras are typically more spiritual. They are considered to be sacred. Affirmations are just what they sound like, statements that affirm that something is true.

Typically you would use an affirmation to create the mental and emotional state that makes you believe that a change has already occurred.

Affirmations are motivational tools to create a new mindset.

You can read affirmations or say them. The best is to do both. If you add a physical component, like using a power pose or jumping up and down, you can turbo charge your results.

Affirmations should always be positive and in the present tense.

You can use the same one every day (think of this as your personal motto) or you can vary them based on your needs. But remember, repetition is what makes this work.

Here are a month's worth (31 to be precise) of my favorite affirmations.

44. Everything is working out for me.

45. I am a winner.

46. The tools I need to succeed are in my possession.

47. My strength is greater than any challenge.

48. I trust the process.

49. I am getting stronger everyday.

50. I am who I want to be.

51. I inspire others.

52. I believe in myself.

53. I dare to be different.

54. I am worthy of love and joy.

55. I am proud of myself and all that I have accomplished.

56. I am enough.

57. I am focused, persistent and will never quit.

58. I am blessed.

59. I am constantly improving.

60. I have a growth mindset.

61. I take responsibility for my life.

62. I have the power to change.

63. I choose to be happy.

64. I love myself unconditionally.

65. I am calm, patient, and in control of my emotions.

66. Every day is filled with new ideas and new possibilities.

67. The money I spend comes back to me multiplied.

68. I control my day.

69. I make a difference.

70. Today is a blessing and a gift.

71. Today I will accomplish great things.

72. I am in love with life.

73. I am open to new opportunities.

74. I am exactly where I need to be.

75. Today is my best day ever.

14 Random Opportunities

When mindfulness becomes a way of life you, don't need to make time to practice. You begin to realize that the opportunity to be present is with you every moment. It's always your choice.

In closing, here are a few golden opportunities that you might not have thought about as ways to create mindful moments. Let's add the following to the list of 90 ways to establish a mindfulness practice in 90 days.

76. Play with a child.

77. Do the dishes.

78. Watch a sunrise.

79. Watch a sunset.

80. Watch the clouds drift by.

81. Play with your pet.

82. Listen to the sounds of nature.

83. Do the dishes.

84. Fold laundry.

85. Garden.

86. Get a massage.

87. Give a massage.

88. Study a work of art.

89. Play a musical instrument.

90. Laugh.

There you have it - 90 ways to make mindfulness a part of your day and a part of your life.

In closing, keep in mind that being mindful is not something that you will ever master. There will always be times when you are spot on and times when your monkey mind is leading the parade.

It's OK.

Always remember that this is a process and that the harder you chase mindfulness the more elusive it becomes.

Be in the moment, and if you don't like the way this one is playing out, don't worry. There's another coming in just another moment.

Actually, isn't the moment already here?

Mindfulness Secrets: 90 Ways In 90 Days

Strategies
1. Decide what area of your life is most in need of your attention.
2. Intentionally create your day.
3. Pick a card to randomly direct your intention.
4. Set alarms and reminders to practice mindfulness.
5. Set a trigger to create awareness.

Techniques

6. Do deep breathing.
7. Be aware of your posture.
8. Practice mindfulness meditation.
9. Do a body scan.
10. Practice square breathing.
11. Study Tai Chi.
12. Do Qigong.
13. Practice Yoga.
14. Make your gym workout more mindful.
15. Go swimming.
16. Take a long walk.
17. Use all of your senses when you eat.
18. Listen to music and focus on different parts and instruments.
19. Become aware of specific colors.
20. Feel textures using different parts of your body.
21. Use smells to create different feelings.

22. Experience things with your eyes closed.
23. Be fully present in your conversations.
24. Give someone a hug of at least 20 seconds.
25. Experience sex with your whole mind and body.
26. Be aware of your thoughts and emotions when you spend money.
27. Be aware of your thoughts and emotions related to your job.
28. Be aware of your thoughts and emotions when you do something charitable.
29. Give everyone you talk to a compliment.
30. See how long you can go without saying anything negative.
31. Spend time being silent.
32. Listen to brain entrainment audios.
33. Use brain monitoring devices.
34. Use mindfulness apps.
35. Put down your smart devices.
36. Pray.
37. Say a mantra.
38. Take a warm shower.
39. Take a cold shower.
40. Float in a sensory deprivation tank.
41. Write about your experiences like they are someone else's.
42. Start a gratitude journal.
43. Do a mind dump by writing down all of your thoughts until you mind is blank.

Daily Affirmations

44. Everything is working out for me.
45. I am a winner.
46. The tools I need to succeed are in my possession.
47. My strength is greater than any challenge.
48. I trust the process.
49. I am getting stronger everyday.
50. I am who I want to be.
51. I inspire others.
52. I believe in myself.
53. I dare to be different.
54. I am worthy of love and joy.
55. I am proud of myself and all that I have accomplished.
56. I am enough.
57. I am focused, persistent and will never quit.
58. I am blessed.
59. I am constantly improving.
60. I have a growth mindset.
61. I take responsibility for my life.
62. I have the power to change.
63. I choose to be happy.
64. I love myself unconditionally.
65. I am calm, patient, and in control of my emotions.
66. Every day is filled with new ideas and new possibilities.
67. The money I spend comes back to me multiplied.

68. I control my day.
69. I make a difference.
70. Today is a blessing and a gift.
71. Today I will accomplish great things.
72. I am in love with life.
73. I am open to new opportunities.
74. I am exactly where I need to be.
75. Today is my best day ever.

Random Opportunities

76. Play with a child.
77. Do the dishes.
78. Watch a sunrise.
79. Watch a sunset.
80. Watch the clouds drift by.
81. Play with your pet.
82. Listen to the sounds of nature.
83. Do the dishes.
84. Fold laundry.
85. Garden.
86. Get a massage.
87. Give a massage.
88. Study a work of art.
89. Play a musical instrument.
90. Laugh.

About The Author

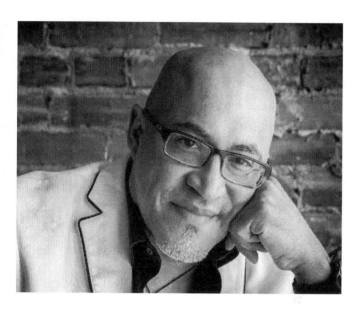

José Johnson has been described as a modern-day renaissance man. José is an internationally recognized martial and energy arts master, having studied various systems of Chinese martial arts, energy arts, mindfulness practices and philosophy for over 30 years. José is also a professional musician, educator, entrepreneur, speaker, writer, consultant and personal mastery coach. José's passion is to empower others to create the transformation that they seek in their lives through an innovative and integrated approach that he calls "Tai Chi for Transformation." This unique approach combines the yin and yang nature of the ancient and the modern; the intellectual and physical; the spiritual and scientific into a unified method for self-development.

José currently is the founder and president of the Personal Mastery and Growth Academy.

You can find him on Facebook, Instagram, YouTube and at coachjosejohnson.com and pmagacademy.com

Made in the USA
Middletown, DE
26 September 2019